Homeopathy & Herbs

HERBS

PRELUDE

It has been the general practice now for some years, when offering means of healing, other than organized medicine, to give or state a disclaimer. . .and the phrasing runs similar to this:

"The material, recipes, botanical materia medica compounds, infusions and decoctions in this book are not intended to replace the services of a physician. A physician should be consulted when the condition logically requires his services."

It has never been brought to my attention that such a statement or disclaimer is required or necessary by law. I would presume that this disclaimer was given to prevent legal action being taken against the author. However, to the best of my knowledge, we still have freedom of the press, and I boldly state that every human being holds an inherent right to select the method of healing or the healer of his choice.

I hold no animosity towards the medical profession. In fact, I respect many members of this profession. But I do not, in the slightest degree, feel that they are the only, nor the best profession in the healing arts.

I am not even slightly convinced that modern medicine, with the thousands of synthetic drugs, has done one iota better in the treatment of disease than the herbalist and his herbs. In fact, it is absolutely true that while many or most drugs are harmful and create side effects (which are often more serious than the disease being treated), the herbalists do not have that problem. I, for one, have never heard of a single instance of serious side effects from the use of recommended herbs by a competent herbalist.

On the other hand, I do not suggest that herbs are the only (or even the best) form of healing. Each individual has the right to read, study, to investigate and then decide on the method or kind of healing that he thinks is best suited to his needs. This inherent right that we have over our body should not be taken lightly. We are indeed "wondrously and fearsomely" made, and everything we do to protect this body will offer great rewards.

INTRODUCTION

The vegetable life of the world has become surrounded by fables, legends and superstitions. The reason for this is probably that to primitive people who symbolized natural phenomena, vegetable like was glorified because it sustained all other life. The tree supplied fuel, house, weapons, boats, as well as food and medicine. Many of these myths form interesting reading but should not form the basis of the use of herbs.

The study of flowers, seeds, roots and barks of plant life has now become a fine science. Much good and useful work has been, and is still being done, by the chemist to discover and extract the active principle of those plants which appear to have an action on the human system. There is, of course, much yet to be done in this direction. We know that a great number of plants used by the herbalist today have a beneficial effect upon the human body in the ailment for which they are recommended, yet in many instances, the reason for the effect is not known. Because of this, some individuals are inclined to scorn the use of herbs. Many of us believe however, that as the chemistry of plants advances, it will be discovered that there is a very good reason for their use and that many will prove superior to the synthetic chemical drugs used today.

It might also be interesting to point out that aspirin, the most widely used drug of all, was originally discovered because natives used an herb containing salicyclic acid as an aid to reduce pain.

To this day, we are not completely sure why salicyclic acid eases pain. The difference between the herb form of salicyclic acid and our new purified, synthetic form should be quite obvious. It is almost impossible to get an overdose if you are chewing the bark of a tree or drinking a tea made from the bark, but with the concentrated tablets, it is an easy thing indeed.

Some may be of a temperament that would abuse the use of herbs - primarily by their overuse. Herbs are Nature's *medicine* - and are to be used as a medicine. They will be of great assistance in time of need, but many of them are capable of upsetting the body chemistry if used over long, protracted periods of time.

The prime requisites of good nutrition, adequate exercise and rest are what keep your resistance to disease up; herbs are used to assist the body in healing itself when a condition of disease has set in. This important principle should be both the indication for and the limitation to the use of herbs.

HERBOLOGY - THE OLDEST HEALING PROFESSION

The history of the use of herbs would be more than ample evidence to substantiate the statement that Herbal Medicine is the fore-runner of all the different forms of healing practiced today. An even closer look at the subject would perhaps give rise to conjecture that a revival of the ancient art of Herbology could save much of the grief and suffering we bear daily from minor complaints which do not warrant going to the doctor.

The premise used so successfully by the practitioner of herbal remedies is that the action of certain herbs, when taken into the body, produces a cleansing, healing activity which then allows the body to normalize its functions and good health ensues. Sound too simple to be true? The basic truths in the entire realm of life are exceedingly simple and also easy to apply, once the understanding is accomplished. In Herbology, the proof is in the pudding, try it - you might like it!

This booklet is designed to begin your knowledge in the possibilities of plant extracts used in a variety of ways to assist the body in its everlasting struggle to maintain health. For many years, the herbal folklore was passed from generation to generation, since the only remedies known were of plant origin. Then the chemist appeared on the scene and through analytical procedures, found what he named the "active" ingredients in these herbal preparations and began the process of "synthesizing" such ingredients so supply could be constant and, perhaps more important, be controlled. It is common knowledge that most drugs today that have stood the test of time are the end product of many months and even years of intensive research to duplicate one of nature's miracle plants which has been helpful in overcoming some complaint of mankind.

HERBAL KNOWLEDGE

The knowledge and the use of herbs should be challenging to every thinking person who is concerned about his health and the health of his or her family.

God has provided a remedy for every disease that might afflict man. Every part of the world has its herbs which are to be used with wisdom in treating disease. Chemical wonder drugs are not the answer to our need, for no drug is without or free from side effects.

Botanicals were created for a purpose, and that purpose should be as clearly understood by us today as it was by the people in past ages, before the chemist came.

It has been said that knowledge is power and he who seeks it is wise and, he who neglects it, does so to his own regret. You have indicated your interest in furthering your knowledge in botanical medicine or herbology by reading this booklet.

Use the information wisely. No one herb can be said to cure any particular condition of the body, but when combined with other complimentary herbs, proper nutrition, rest, and good living habits, amazing results occur.

A pattern of living emerges which is preventive in nature, not emergency treatment. It will only be through this method that a strong nation will once again emerge. It is the exception today, rather than the rule, to meet a truly well person. We have strayed from Nature's Principles and search impotently for a chemical panacea. It will never be found!

Our bodies are equipped with everything to prevent illness and disease. But that equipment breaks down when we abuse and neglect it by improper food, exercise and the excessive consumption of coffee, tea, alcohol and tobacco.

Herbs are capable of assisting the body to return to normal function. But don't expect miracles overnight. Nature works slowly in her rebuilding processes, just as a skilled craftsman does not proceed in a haphazard manner. It is often necessary to clean out the debris of disease before healing can take place. Your patience will be rewarded!

A lack of knowledge based on truth is accountable for much of the suffering and misery of humanity. A practical knowledge of herbology can save money, suffering and even premature death.

DEFINITION

To properly define an herb, one should bear in mind that this category includes all such items of vegetable origin that will serve as medicinal remedies for internal and external purposes. Some will have specific healing properties, some will help to maintain health, others can be used as preventatives, while still others may be of special benefit in furthering the recovery from an ailment. By these actions, herbs become helpful in cleaning up the blood stream, liver, kidneys, the nervous system, and other organs - and do this without side effects that the drugs in such common use today have.

The question has often been asked, "If many drugs used today are really synthetic active factors of herbs, they why are they harmful?" We should recognize that many drugs can have a place in emergency situations, it is the indiscriminate use of them in a concentrated form without their natural synergist such as are found in herbs, that create problems for many. The old saying, "An ounce of prevention is worth a pound of cure," is certainly applicable in the field of Herbology. The student who recognized the properties of herbs and then applies that knowledge to his own body, can often prevent serious illness and degenerative disease within himself.

HERB CLASSIFICATION

You should be encouraged to read some of the many good texts on Herbology, which are far more complete and detailed than this work is intended. But, in order to facilitate your study, you should be familiar with the peculiar terminology used by Herbalists.

Anodyne	capable of relieving pain
Antihelminthic	capable of expelling worms
Antiphlogistic	capable of relieving inflammation
Antispasmodic	capable of relieving spasms
Aperient	mildly laxative
Aphrodisiac	capable of stimulating sexual desire
Carminative	capable of removing gases from the gastrointestinal tract
Cathartic	a active purgative, a harsh laxative
Demulcent	capable of soothing mucus membranes, particularly of gastrointestinal tract and lungs
Diaphoretic	capable of increasing perspiration
Diuretic	capable of inducing urination
Emetic	capable of inducing vomiting
Expectorant	capable of facilitating the removal of mucus from the lungs
Hemostatic	capable of slowing down or stopping hemorrhage
Hypnotic	capable of inducing sleep
Irritant	capable of producing local

	inflammatory reactions
Nervine	capable of acting as a sedative for for nerves
Oxytoxic	capable of stimulating uterine contractions
Stomachic	capable of increasing function of the stomach
Sudorific	capable of inducing perspiration
Tonic	capable of increasing strength
Vermifuge	capable of expelling parasites
Vulnerary	used to heal wounds

HERBAL PREPARATION TERMS

INFUSION - Pour one pint of boiling water over one ounce of herb and let stand for 1/2 hour. Strain clear liquid off. Dose is one tablespoonful to one ounce three times daily.

DECOCTION - Pour 1 1/2 pints cold water over one ounce of herb and boil for 20 to 30 minutes. Strain clear liquid off. Dose is one tablespoonful to one ounce three times daily.

TINCTURE - Prepared by use of alcohol to extract the active ingredient from the herb. Usually 1 to 2 ounces of herb are steeped in 1 pint of alcohol for several days with frequent shaking of the ingredients daily. This is then strained and 1 tablespoonful used three times daily. (Vodka is the favorite form of easily obtained ethyl alcohol.)

CAPSULE - Almost any herb can be powdered and then encapsulated in a two piece hardshell gelatin capsule. This offers a wide variety of uses, such as adding to hot water for tea, making a paste for poultices, for making a tincture, decoction, or infusion, or for swallowing intact.

TABLET - Almost any herb can be tableted. This means of preparation offers most of the advantages of the capsule at a more reasonable price.

Please note that the instructions give earlier are very general in nature and do not apply in every instance. For example, some tinctures may be used in such small amounts that 5 or 6 drops would be sufficient.

HERBS IN COMMON USE

The following is not a total list of all the herbs available, but is a partial list of some of the more commonly used ones, with some interesting facts about each one and historical uses for the herb. Since herbs have been used since the beginning of our world for medicinal purposes, you may wish to try such a natural approach to body normalization, and have a lot of fun in doing so!

ALFALFA - One of the best of all the herbs, alfalfa is readily available and has a history of offering dramatic benefit to its users. A great deal is known about alfalfa, probably because of the work of Dr. Benjamin Ershoff, who conducted extensive experimental work on the effect of alfalfa supplementation in animal diets. It is an excellent source of trace mineral nutrients and has *diuretic*, *tonic* and *nervine* properties. It has also been used by many for the relief of the symptoms of arthritis.

BILBERRY LEAVES - The leaves of this plant contain a glucoquinine which helps to lower blood sugar levels in diabetics. The plant grows quite freely in the northwestern states and is commonly referred to as the Huckleberry or Whortleberry. In general, the properties are *astringent*, *tonic*, *hypoglycemic*, *antiseptic* and *antidiarrheal*. The hypoglycemic properties are not to be interpreted as an indication for those who have hypoglycemia to not use it. As in so many of the natural remedies, the effect of this herb is more normalizing, and tends to reduce the high blood sugar levels of the diabetic rather than producing hypoglycemia. A tea made of the leaves is especially effective in diarrhea. This action probably results from its astringent and antiseptic properties. Also, these same properties make the tea an excellent remedy for canker sores, as a gargle or mouthwash and as an external application for skin problems.

BLACK COHOSH - Native to the U.S. and also called black snakeroot, squaw root and bugbane. An herb of many uses, Black Cohosh is usefully employed as a remedy in dropsy, hysteria, and various afflictions of the lungs. It is used widely by women in menopause, where it seems to have a pronounced calming effect. The major properties are *nervine*, *diuretic*, and *antispasmodic*. It is said that Black Cohosh is a wonderful remedy for high blood pressure.

BLESSED THISTLE - Generally classified as a bitter herb, this botanical is cultivated widely in Europe for its medicinal properties. It is considered a *febrifuge* (capable of reducing fever), a *diaphoretic*, a *vulnerary*, a *tonic*, and a *stimulant*. As you can see, these properties are very compatible and assist in making this herb very valuable in problems involving flu or colds. Many herbalists, in addition to the above properties, feel that this herb is specific in promoting the flow of bile and in purifying the liver. Its natural habitat is primarily Southern Europe and Western Asia; the whole herb is used in making powdered preparations or liquid extracts.

BLUEBERRY LEAVES - This plant belongs to the same family as the afore-mentioned Bilberry and, therefore, has the same *astringent*, *tonic, hypoglycemic*, *antiseptic*, and *antidiarrheal* properties. Its use would also be identical.

BLUE VERVAIN - This is an excellent *sudorific* or *diaphoretic* herb. It will induce an opening of the pores allowing toxins to be excreted from the body. This action creates the reputation this herb has as a *febrifuge* or fever reducing herb. It also has *diuretic* properties and is mildly stimulating. It is my opinion that this herb is not adequately known or respected, but by those who use it, the rewards will be great. Its habitat is throughout all of Europe and is quite commonly seen as a flowering "volunteer" beside roadways and in meadows. The whole herb is used for botanical preparations.

BUCHU - This herb is used mostly for chronic or acute

problems of the genito-urinary tract, such as cystitis, pyelitis, urethritis, and prostatitis. It has also been used for bladder gravel and leucorrhea. Extremely helpful as a *diuretic*.

BUCKTHORN BARK - Again we have one of Nature's wonders in this wonderful herb. It contains certain substances which, after digestion, are absorbed in the blood stream and have a stimulating effect on the bile. In fact, while they stimulate the flow of bile, they, at the same time, combine with the bile and are soon discharged back into the intestinal tract. Since bile is Nature's laxative, this soon produces very easy movement of the bowels. Buckthorn does not gripe as does senna, which is undigestable for the most part and acts as an irritant. This herb also contains a compound which has a calming effect on the gastrointestinal tract, thus it can be used for extended periods of time without discomfort. Buckthorn bark is primarily a *chologogue* and a mild *purgative*.

CALENDULA - An herb which was used widely and valued highly in days gone by. It was used as a tincture, an ointment and internally as a powder. It contains an excellent essential oil containing carotenoid (carotene, calenduline, and lycopine). It is considered one of the most *vulnerary* herbs available, encouraging the rapid healing of both external wounds and internal irritations. Another property is its *antiphlogistic* action which assists in relieving inflammations. It is thus quite easily seen why Calendula had a reputation in the treatment of ulcers, stomach cramps, colitis, diarrhea and other gastrointestinal irritations.

CATNIP - Also known as catmint, this herb has many properties including *relaxant*, *diaphoretic*, *carminative*, *anodyne*, and *nervine*. The leaves of catnip are used in preparing the remedies and are gathered sometimes twice a year - the plant is so sturdy and vigorous. The most common uses are for upset stomach and diarrhea such as might be associated with the flu, and for vague aches and pains which might also be associated with the flu. Although this herb is a native of Europe and Asia, its medicinal properties were so well thought of, that it was brought over to America by immigrants, and because of its hearty characteristics, grew abundantly in practically all areas.

CAYENNE - Also known as African Bird Pepper. An extremely popular herb, cayenne has properties of equalizing circulation, which is very important in healing of any nature. Also because of this effect on the circulation, cayenne (capsicum) can be of assistance to those who suffer from cold extremities. Very useful in all inflammations, stomach and bowel disorders, fevers, pleurisy, and may be used externally as a poultice or ingredient in a liniment for sprains, etc. Considered a *stomachic*, *carminative*, *demulcent*, *tonic*, and *antiphlogistic*.

CHAMOMILE - This herb is probably best know for its action as a remedy for nervous conditions of women, particularly during the menstrual time. It is used to relieve a congested uterus and stimulating the menstrual flow. A poultice applied to swollen tissue is helpful in reducing both pain and swelling. Classified as *nervine* and *emmenagogue*.

CHAPARRAL - This herb was brought into prominence recently when certain individuals reported anticancer activity from its use and two universities began studies on Chaparral. Whatever the outcome of such studies, Chaparral is an effective *blood cleanser and purifier* of the whole body.

CHICKWEED - Although there are many uses for this herb, I have found that one of its most salutary properties is that of an appetite depressant. Many are the stories I have heard from individuals on diets who were having trouble with a powerful appetite. When I recommended Chickweed tea for this strong desire for food, the response was almost always the same - "It's gone." Other uses for this herb are: *demulcent*, *emollient*, *anodyne*. In homeopathic medicine, this herb is used to relieve rheumatic pains and psoriasis. It can be used in a liniment form for aches and pains. Some also consider Chickweed as an excellent herbal remedy for pulmonary complaints. The whole herb is used.

CINCHONA BARK - An herb which comes to us from South America, Cinchona owes its properties to many alkaloids, including quinine, quinidine, cinchonine and cinchonidine. These alkaloids can act as powerful *astringents* and *febrifuges*. The herb is cultivated in America, Asia and part of Africa where soil and climate are suitable for growth. The bark of the tree and roots are used in botanical medicine for fevers and malaria, as a preventive for influenza and as a *stomachic*. A very effective herb, particularly when used in combination with others.

COMFREY - It would be difficult to name a more useful herb. It is a soothing *demulcent*, mitigating irritations of the gastrointestinal tract and bronchi. Also acts as an *expectorant* and can be used as a *poultice*.

CORN SILK - Medicinal properties are dependent upon the oil contained within the Corn Silk, therefore, keep the storage container tightly closed to prevent oxidation. Considered a valuable remedy in many urinary and bladder conditions. A soothing *demulcent* and a *tonic diuretic*.

CRAMPBARK - A time honored *relaxant* to the uterus and ovaries. Useful in uterine cramps, it can prevent miscarriage due to such premature cramping. Acts as an *antispasmodic*.

DAMIANA - Although this herb is said to encourage pleasant, amorous dreams, it is probably more useful as a *tonic* to the nervous problems of menopausal women.

DANDELION - Possibly one of the most hated herbs (by gardeners) which exists. On the other hand, it is also one of the finest herbs for general use. Dandelion is one of the very best herbs known for inducing the flow of bile from the liver. It can be so effective that the first stages of cirrhosis of the liver can be alleviated by consistent use. Such stimulation of liver function has many beneficial results. Edema can be relieved if related to liver problems; diabetes recovery is enhanced with a normal functioning liver, and all forms of toxins are eliminated. Dandelion is a *chologogue*, tonic, a *stimulant* and a *diuretic.*

FENNEL - The primary part of this herb used are the seeds. Its main use is as a *stomachic* and *carminative*, although is has *diuretic* properties. Fennel helps to relieve colic, abdominal cramps, flatulence and also to expel mucus secretions from the gastrointestinal tract. It is also used to loosen mucus from persistent coughs. It can be diluted and used as an eyewash to relieve strain and irritation. Fennel is grown commercially for the most part, although certain areas find it in quite plentiful supply growing wild. Its medicinal value probably comes from a very bitter, acrid essential oil contained in the seeds.

FENUGREEK - A pleasant, fragrant herb often used as a tea to assist in expelling mucus and phlegm from the bronchial tubes. Also used for sore throats and as a poultice for wounds. *Expectorant.*

GARLIC - This herb has been used for so long, for so many different conditions, by so many different people, and is so effective, that a book could be written about it alone. Common uses are as an *antihelminthic*, *carminative*, *diaphoretic*, *stomachic*, *antiseptic*, and *diuretic*. It is also used to assist in lowering blood pressure.

GINGER - Although Ginger is normally thought of as a

culinary herb, it falls in the same category as garlic - in that it has powerful medicinal qualities. Many of these properties are beneficial in preparing foods - the *carminative*, *appetite stimulant*, and *stomachic* effect can certainly be applied to a variety of otherwise dull foods. However, one of its greatest traits lies in its *systemic cleansing* effect both through the normal channels of the bowels and kidneys, but also through the skin. The *diaphoretic* action is very useful in the herbalist's hands for any number of conditions, including colds, diabetes, and any toxic condition. The rootstalk is the part used for powders and tinctures.

GINSENG - The Chinese use Ginseng as a preventive for any number of disorders. It is commonly used for its *tonic* properties and is considered an *aphrodisiac* and *stimulant*. Appears to have some effect on the pituitary and adrenal glands.

GOLDENSEAL - Also known as Yellow Paint Root, Orange Root, Ground Raspberry, Yellow Indian Paint, Turmeric Root, Jaundice Root. Considered by some to be the single finest herb available. It acts so well as a blood purifier, that certain drugs are completely removed from the body within hours of taking it when they normally would be present for days. It is useful as a *blood purifier* and an *antiseptic*, and *tonic* for the digestive tract and mucous membranes. Can be used as a mouthwash or gargle, externally for wounds or sores, and internally as a liver tonic.

HAWTHORN BERRY - Books have been written about

this single herb which should give one some idea of its effectiveness. It is often a mystery to herbalists why the drug industry overlooks a proven remedy that is so readily available. Hawthorn is a strong *cardiac tonic* and helps in both high and low blood pressure. Tachycardia and arrhythmia also respond well to this herb since it is both *antispasmodic* and *sedative*.

Hawthorn has also been used in treating insomnia of nervous origin. Herbalists also use it as a *vasodilator* and this probably explains its action in treating high blood pressure since the relaxing of the blood vessels will lower pressure. It is good for heart muscles weakened by age, for inflammation of the heart muscle, has been used for arteriosclerosis, and is highly recommended for all executives under stress.

HOPS FLOWERS - An excellent *nervine*, *anodyne*, and *sedative*. It has been used in dysmenorrhea, rheumatism, and neuralgia. It is said that hops flowers are an effective herb for insomnia.

HORSETAIL - There are few herbs that equal Horsetail as a *diuretic*, *astringent*, or *hemostatic*. Its use is known back in the early centuries when it was used as a mouthwash and gargle for mouth and throat infections. Herbalists use it extensively for inducing the flow of urine, for healing and normalizing irritations in cystitis and other bladder and urethral tract problems. The hemostatic property for internal bleeding has also been well established and used. As a plant, horsetail prefers dry, rocky ground but grows very well in its chosen habitat. Its therapeutic use has been known since before the 16th century; currently respect for it is growing rather than subsiding.

HYSSOP - This bushy, evergreen plant was once very widely cultivated for medicinal purposes but has recently found favor as an ornamental shrub. Hyssop is best known in the herbal field for its *astringent*, *expectorant*, *stimulant* and *tonic* properties. It can also be used as a *carminative* and *stomachic* which makes it an ideal herb for use in all types of lung congestions with upset stomach including, but not limited to, the flu. Some would say that Hyssop has secondary properties of inducing perspiration (*diaphoretic*) and diuresis (*diuretic*), but these only substantiate the other properties and enhance the elimination of toxic waste products from the body. Under certain circumstances, it could be said that Hyssop has *febrifuge* (fever reducing) properties.

JUNIPER - The berries of this herb have long been used as a *diuretic*. Its use in a variety of kidney and bladder problems has withstood the test of time.

LADY'S SLIPPER - This particular herb expends all of its medicinal properties on the nervous system, therefore, it is a *nervine* of first importance. Restlessness, insomnia and menstrual irritability respond well to this herb.

LAVENDER FLOWERS - Apart from having a delightful fragrance, Lavender Flowers are an effective and valued medicinal herb. The flowers are the most commonly used, but in some parts of the world, the leaves are also used in making tinctures, decoctions, etc. Perhaps its most effective use is in a tincture where the oil is distilled from the herb. Lavender Flowers are used as *antispasmodics*, *sedatives*, and a mild *diuretic*. They have been used for headaches, fainting, nervous prostration, and dizziness. The leaves have *stomachic*, *carminative* and *chologogue* properties. These are usually used as a tea for flatulence, nausea and vomiting.

LICORICE - An old and very popular remedy. It is often used in conditions of the mucous membranes of the throat, but perhaps the most dramatic results come from the effect it has on the adrenal glands. A *tonic*, **demulcent**, and *expectorant*.

LOBELIA - A powerful *emetic*, Lobelia is also used as a *nervine*, *antispasmodic*, *expectorant*, and a great equalizer of the circulation. Some consider it a specific remedy for asthma. Some herbalists state, "We believe that Lobelia is one of the finest remedies with which a kind Providence has blessed mankind."

MANDRAKE - A favorite Indian remedy, Mandrake assists in cleansing the liver, while at the same time acting as a *cathartic*. Moderate doses offer the benefits of cleansing, without the catharsis.

MARSHMALLOW - This herb would probably wither away with mortification if it knew what most people associate its name with. The whipped sugar confection of today contains none of this herb and is a nutritional folly. The most efficacious part of the Marshmallow herb is the root, although the leaves and flowers are also used. It is one of the best *demulcents* available and also is an *emollient*, *mucilaginous*, mild *diuretic*, *protective* and *vulnerary*. Marshmallow is very soothing and healing to the inflamed respiratory, alimentary, intestinal, and genitourinary systems. Its diuretic and demulcent qualities are especially useful for urinary and prostate complaints because it has no astringent action and is quite relaxing. It is soothing and healing to all mucous membranes so, it is a very valuable herb in the botanical medicine world.

MILFOIL - This herb is found the world over and has a long history of application as a healing agent. It is considered an *antispasmodic*, a *carminative*, and a nerve *tonic*. Since certain temporary (we hope) restrictions have been imposed on mistletoe, many herbalists will use Milfoil as a very able substitute. This is another blessing in using herbs. Many have similar functions and properties so may be substituted freely as supply dictates. Milfoil is excellent for excitable or cramping muscles, for poor appetite or upset stomach, and general nervousness.

MISTLETOE - An ancient remedy, replete with folklore, Mistletoe is classified as a *nervine*, with some literature naming it as a specific for epilepsy. The FDA considers this herb a drug and not safe for general use.

MULLEIN - A hardy herb which grows naturally from the Atlantic Coast to the Rocky Mountains. It is used as an *anodyne*, a fabulous *demulcent*, an *expectorant*, an *antispasmodic*, and a mild *diuretic*. Mullein makes an excellent remedy for coughs, colds, hoarseness, bronchitis, and catarrh. It does help to relieve pain and induce relaxation. Herbalists have said of Mullein that it is the best pain killer in the entire kingdom and has no side effects or harm. This is the reason that when a fever rages or a respiratory inflammation causes a great deal of stress, Mullein is an excellent remedy to use with other herbs since it quietens one down and allows the healing process to take place.

MYRR GUM - A *carminative*, *stomachic*, and *antiseptic* herb, Myrr Gum is often overlooked by the users of herbs. It has *astringent* properties and is particularly effective anywhere inflammation, soreness, or wounds are present.

PARSLEY - This herb is an excellent remedy for retained or difficult urination, acting primarily as a *diuretic*. A hot fomentation applied to insect bites brings instant relief. Reputed to be of benefit in gall bladder problems also.

PASSION FLOWER - Very often used in medicines as an ingredient. This emphasizes the effective results that Passion Flower produces. It is an excellent *antispasmodic* and *sedative*. It is also an effective *diaphoretic*. These properties make is very useful in heart conditions, nervousness, insomnia, hysteria, and other neuro-muscular disorders. Some herbalists consider it a great replacement for tranquilizers, particularly in combination with some of the other nervines.

PEPPERMINT - Possibly one of the most common of all the herbs, being used for centuries as a *stomachic* and *carminative* herb. An excellent remedy for colic, gas on the stomach, nausea, vomiting, diarrhea, dysentery and influenza. Can be applied externally for aches and pains. A hot cup of Peppermint tea will bring a natural warmth to the whole system, and is both relaxing and restorative.

PLEURISY ROOT - As the name implies, this herb is used in such chest and lung troubles as bronchitis, asthma, chronic cough, acute catarrh, pneumonia, pleurisy, croup, and colds. It acts as an *expectorant*, a *sudorific*, and a *diaphoretic*.

POKE ROOT - A native North American herb, this herb is commonly used for its *laxative* properties. It also has *anodyne* properties and seems to have an appetite inhibiting effect that could be very beneficial in weight reducing programs. The root of the herb is most often used, although the berries and sometimes the leaves have been used.

QUASSIA - Also known as Bitter Bark, Bitter Ash, Bitter Wood. This herb acts as a general *tonic*, and has been used to help reduce the desire for alcoholic beverages. It acts as a *febrifuge*, helping to reduce fever, and is well known for its *antihelminthic* properties, and expelling parasites from the intestinal tract.

RED RASPBERRY - A very effective herb for female problems. It decreases an excessive menstrual flow without stopping it. Red Raspberry is recommended for pregnant women, making delivery easier and the possibility of hemorrhage less. It relieves after-birth pains and assists milk secretion. An *antiemetic*, *astringent*, *tonic*, and *stomachic*.

RED SAGE - An herb of many properties, Red Sage is classified as a *diuretic*, *stimulant*, *tonic*, *diaphoretic*, *stomachic*, and *astringent*. An herb with so many medicinal effects, it is often used as part of a general cleansing program.

SARSAPARILLA - Often used as an herbal beverage, Sarsaparilla also is said to stimulate the action of estrogen in females. Probably for this reason, it is classified as an *aphrodisiac*, although it may be a better blood purifier than a tonic.

SKULLCAP - Also known as Hoodwart, Hooded Willow Herb, Mad Dogwood, Mad Weed, Helmet Flower. This is one of the very best nerve tonics, and is very quietening and soothing to the nerves. Promotes sleep for the insomniac and even makes aches and pains more bearable. A powerful *nervine*, *antispasmodic*, and *tonic*.

SLIPPERY ELM - This herb has long held a reputation of soothing and healing the mucous membranes of the lungs and gastrointestinal tract. It is a *demulcent* of the first order, so in addition to the above areas, it is also suggested in problems of the urinary tract and bowels.

SQUAW VINE - Also known as Partridge Berry,

Checkerberry, Deerberry, Winter Clover, Hive Vine. An herb considered to be an excellent medicine to take during pregnancy and is claimed to make childbirth easier. This herb was held in high regard by Indian women who used it during pregnancy, for uterine problems, urinary tract problems such as leukorrhea, etc. Considered a *diuretic*, an *astringent*, a *tonic*, and an *alterative*.

THYME - An old time remedy, thyme can be used freely. Excellent when used as a hot tea, inducing profuse perspiration. Safe for children - small doses given frequently produce excellent results. A household remedy of good repute, thyme is used in lung afflictions to induce perspiration and relax the nerves.
A *sudorific*, *nervine*, and *antispasmodic*.

UVA URSI - Also known as Bearberry, Upland Cranberry, Kinikinnic, Wild Cranberry, Mealberry. Very useful in all kidney troubles, mucus discharges with pus and blood from the bladder. A specific in kidney, bladder and urinary problems. Uva Ursi acts as a *diuretic*, *astringent* and *tonic*.

VALERIAN - Also known as Vandal Root and All Heal. Excellent nerve tonic, useful in hysterics. Good for convulsions in children, and helps to soothe a bloated stomach. Especially useful in nervous conditions, this herb can be used for restful sleep by any age. An excellent *nervine*, Valerian also has an *antispasmodic* effect.

WALNUT LEAVES - The leaves of the Black Walnut tree offer *vermifuge* properties as well as being *astringent* in nature.

YARROW - Sometimes confused with Milfoil, true Yarrow is a distinct herb. It is used as a *diaphoretic*, *astringent*, *diuretic*, *tonic*, *vulnerary*, and a mild *antispasmodic*. It opens the pores freely with its relaxing action on the skin, and with its perspiration inducing properties, tends to clear the blood of its morbid waste materials. It has a primary effect on fevers, all types of eruptive disorders such as measles, chicken pox, etc., and also helps to regulate and control liver function. The whole herb, as well as the flowers, are used in making medicinal extracts.

YERBA SANTA - Also known as Consumption Weed, Gum Plant, Bear's Weed, Tar Weed and Mountain Balm. This is a well tried and much used remedy in chronic laryngitis, bronchitis and various lung problems. Effective where there is an excessive discharge from the nose. An excellent *tonic* and *expectorant* in all lung problems.

PRACTICAL APPLICATIONS

In the past pages, we have reviewed several of the more effective and easily obtained herbs. But, just like most other plants on this earth, herbs seem to work better when in combination with similar acting herbs. It is my opinion that the combination of several herbs relieves one of the possibilities of error in judgement which is inherent in the use of single herb.

In this section, I will outline areas of the body which can be effectively assisted in a return to normal function by the use of herbal combinations. It is important to remember that herbs must be dissolved in order to be most effective - this is no problem when used as a tea, but when talking them in capsule or tablet form, it is wise to swallow them with a full glass of water, preferably sipped over a period of five minutes.

Many times, the addition of vitamins, minerals or glandular extracts to an herbal formula potentates the results severalfold. This synergistic effect which occurs can both decrease the total amount and the time required for desired effect. Most of the formulae are designed to be taken twice daily, usually two tablets or capsules at a time.

GASTROINTESTINAL - Ulcers, gastritis, heartburn, indigestion, colitis, diverticulitis.

Comfrey Leaf	Cayenne Pepper
Myrrh Gum	Peppermint
Calcium Carbonate	Pectin

GENERAL CLEANSING - High blood pressure, chronic infections, chronic degenerative disease, headaches, allergies, arthritis, rheumatism, overweight.

Garlic	Chaparral
Quassia	Fenugreek
Black Cohosh	Red Sage
Goldenseal	

RESPIRATORY - Bronchitis, mucus and phlegm accumulation, chronic cough, pneumonia, pleurisy, asthma, emphysema.

Slippery Elm	Fenugreek
Thyme	Pleurisy Root
Lobelia	Yerba Santa
Vitamin A	Vitamin C

FEMALE DISORDERS - Amenorrhea, dysmenorrhea, cramps, discharge, menopause.

Red Raspberry	Squaw Vine
Damiana	Sarsaparilla
Cramp Bark	Black Cohosh
Licorice	Ginseng
Vitamin E	Calcium

NERVOUS DISORDERS - Restlessness, insomnia, hyperirritability, hysteria, depression, worry, nervous headaches.

Valerian	Hops Flowers
Lady's Slipper	Chamomile
Lobelia	Tryptophan
Skullcap	

KIDNEY DISORDERS - Kidney stones, bladder gravel, burning on urination, difficult urination, edema, frequency of urination, low back pains because of poor kidney function, cystitis.

Alfalfa	Buchu
Juniper	Parsley
Uva Ursi	Corn Silk
Magnesium	Vitamin A

VERMIFUGE - Worms, parasites.

- Garlic
- Black Walnut Leaves
- Mandrake
- Quassia

HERBAL FORMULATIONS

It has been my experience that herbs work better when combined with other herbs that are synergistic and compatible in their use and effect. In line with the work in which I gave several combination formulations for different applications, the following formulations are representative of the combinations of herbs I would use for general conditions.

DIABETES

- Chaparral
- Ginger
- Blueberry Leaves
- Dandelion Root
- Goldenseal
- Bilberry Leaves
- Walnut Leaves
- Chromium
- Vanadium

FEVER

- Blue Vervain
- Comfrey
- Buckthorn Bark
- Chamomile
- Cinchona Bark
- Yarrow
- Yarrow Flowers

FLU

- Yarrow
- Chamomile
- Pleurisy Root
- Blessed Thistle
- Catnip
- Hyssop

PROSTATE

- Cayenne
- Marshmallow
- Goldenseal
- Ginger
- Juniper Berry
- Prostate Extract
- Zinc

APPETITE
(depressant)
Poke Root
Chickweed
Fennel
Riboflavin
Phenylalanine

HEART

Hawthorn Berry
Valerian
Peppermint
Passion Flower
Cayenne
Heart Extract

SORE THROAT
Slippery Elm
Cayenne
Peppermint
Chaparral

COUGHS
Mullein
Chamomile
Buckthorn Bark
Comfrey
Yerba Santa
Cinchona

LOZENGE - Many do not associate herbs with cough drops or lozenges but, they can be very effective ingredients. Here is an example of an herbal combination that will provide mucilaginous, soothing effect while at the same time provide a healing atmosphere.

Slippery Elm Bark
Gum Acacia
Sorbitol
Peppermint
Cayenne

COMFREY-PEPSIN - This formula is a combination herbal and digestive combination which was popularized by Dr. William D. Kelly, who uses it to dissolve the mucus film which coats the small intestine in many individuals. When this occurs, nutrients cannot get through the intestinal wall properly and, therefore, are not absorbed into the blood stream.

The formula I suggest is:
Comfrey..................... 300 mg
Pepsin .... 100 mg
Wheat Germ .... 100 mg

NOTE: The foregoing dietary recommendations are for general nutritional purposes only, and are not to be considered substitutes for any specific nutritional counsel or advise of your doctor concerning specific situations. Certain persons considered experts may disagree with one or more of the preceding statements or recommendations.

THE CREATIVE RESTORATION DIET

This message is for you! It is a health program designed for modern living with a great deal of study and practical clinical experience resulting in this concise and precision engineered schedule. Any program can only be as effective as its application. Anything worth doing is worth doing well, so why not make it a real challenge to put it to work for a mere 30 days of your life - and in return have a chance at increased health, the greatest gift of all!!

INCOMPATIBLE WITH THIS PROGRAM

Certain Habits are incompatible with your search for health. You cannot build with one hand while tearing down with the other and expect to fashion a monument. The following are incompatible with good health:

1. **Consumption of alcohol.** This has been proven

scientifically to destroy the brain as well as liver cells.

2. **Smoking.** So much evidence has been presented, we need not elaborate, but specifically it is carcinogenic and destroys Vitamin C.

3. **Over-consumption of coffee and tea.** Both of these contain habit-forming drugs and are deleterious to the central nervous system. You may substitute herb teas or cereal beverages (available at health food stores).

UNDERSTANDING THE CREATIVE RESTORATION DIET

This is a recommended method of eating foods to induce you to "automatically" improve your diet. **IT MUST BE UNDERSTOOD**, not just blindly followed. You must learn to lead your own way. Unlike the dull, restricted menu-type diet which requires discipline to enforce, this educational approach can be interesting. It encourages a greater, rather than lesser, variety of foods, thus both taste and appetite are more likely to be satisfied. There is also a great satisfaction in being able to select foods by reason of good judgement and common sense, rather than by the usual hit or miss method.

Therefore, please read the following information carefully. If you understand why you are asked to follow certain rules and guidelines, it will be much easier to gain your cooperation. It merely takes plain, common sense and a wisp of willpower. Your conscience should become your guide. Since this diet consists primarily of vegetables, meat, cheese, fish, poultry, and fruit, it is high in minerals, especially potassium, an essential mineral of prime importance in the body chemistry. Because it is high in fiber foods, which are both cleansing and speed up the tract time, it encourages a favorable intestinal environment. It is intended to eliminate a high proportion of so called "empty calorie" foods, so it should have an excellent **weight normalization** influence.

Naturally, all of the foods which one should not eat cannot be mentioned. Only the major classifications are mentioned in this regard, listing a few categories only. The guidelines for food combinations are few and easy to follow. Emphasis is placed upon the positive "what to eat" nature of dieting. It is a diet you can believe in because it is deemed to be right, founded in truth, rather than fancy or statistics. **Basic rules to follow are listed at the end of the text. These should be learned and practiced until they become matters of habit.**

Regarding White Flour and White Sugar Products

Not only are white flour and sugar products devoid of their natural occurring vitamins and minerals, but the less desirable calories are concentrated until they become little more than pure starch and carbohydrate.

Why is this abuse of Nature's stores brought about? In the case of white flour, shelf-life is the main reason. All commercial white flour is processed so that it can be stored for long periods of time. To make this possible, most of the "life" is removed from the whole wheat berries. Since the oil is removed, it cannot turn rancid. Everything subject to oxidation has been removed. If it were not so, spoilage would be very rapid, often within a period of a few days.

White sugar is refined for another reason. In its liquid form as a cane juice, it would ferment rapidly and would require refrigeration from can field to user. Obviously, this would not serve commercial purposes. Granulated sugar did! But the attendant loss of vitamins and minerals, plus the intensive concentration of purified carbohydrate, made a mixture too rich to handle by your body, much like the carburetor on your car when too much gas is mixed with the air.

An important feature of the Creative Restoration Diet is to eat maximum quantities of live foods and eliminate purified foods. White flour products and white sugar products are dead foods (no enzymes and most or all of the vitamins and minerals removed) and are purified substances which the body finds difficult to adapt to normal metabolism.

It is comparatively simple to eliminate much white sugar from the diet simply by not eating candy, pastries and so forth, made from white sugar. However, many find it difficult to eliminate all white flour products such as bread, bakery rolls and, pasta foods (macaroni, spaghetti, pizza and the like). The elimination of white flour products is essential, however, if the fullest benefits are to be obtained from the Creative Restoration Diet.

Regarding the Use of Uncooked Foods - Let's look at your diet from the aspect of how much of it consists of uncooked or raw foods. Many people go to one extreme with no more raw food than a smattering of lettuce or an occasional glass of fruit juice. The remainder of their diet is completely cooked! **The eating of fresh, raw foods daily should never be left to chance.** Two outstanding all-season foods are recommended as always available: 1.Tomatoes and Tomato Juice; 2. Raw Cabbage.

Although raw tomatoes are usually best, canned tomatoes, without preservatives added, are on the list of acceptable foods. Tomatoes are one of the few vegetables which lend themselves well to the canning process. In fact, tomatoes canned at the height of their natural perfection, are higher in food value than the hot house varieties sold in off-season. The same applies to tomato juice, with both offering rich sources of potassium and vitamins A, B, and C.

Salads made with raw cabbage instead of lettuce can be one of the greatest taste surprises you have ever had. Cabbage in raw form is one of our richest sources of essential vitamins and minerals. It stores well, if not better, than any other raw food, keeping its nutrients beneath its protective wrapper in the leaves. **It is indispensable to the success of this diet, that a high quality raw food be included in the diet daily.** Tomato and cabbage have been suggested - if at all possible, I use one cupful of raw cabbage with a little raw potato or jicima or water chestnut mixed in every day. Raw carrots, cauliflower, sprouts, celery, etc. are almost always available and can be used to excellent advantage.

Regarding Use of Meat Products - Meats, such as veal, beef, lamb, and chicken are good sources of protein. However, even though the protein intake in adequate, insofar as quantity is concerned, quality is an even more important point to consider. Incomplete proteins leave out pieces of the "building block" mechanism, and like a jigsaw puzzle with pieces missing, the whole picture suffers. This can be a good reason to supplement the diet with a multi-source protein product to assure an adequate amino acid supply and balance.

Also in regard to protein ingestion, its breakdown into amino acids is essential to its utilization. This is called the process of digestion. If digestion fails to liquefy the meat (protein), spoilage can occur in the intestinal tract - a process called putrefaction. Effects of putrefaction in the gastrointestinal tract are bad breath, foul odored stool and a general decrease in energy. This is good reason to supplement the diet with an appropriate enzyme product, both facilitating breakdown of the protein and preventing putrefaction.

Contrary to some opinions, the grinding of meat into small particles, e.g., hamburger, does not increase its digestability. Indeed, grinding of meat can have deleterious effects. Ground meat spoils rapidly at room temperature, whole meat does not, in fact, aging of whole meat can make it more tender by a sort of "predigestion" which occurs.

It is postulated that nucleic acids are released when meat is ground, coming out with the meat juices, apparently making spoilage very fast by this means. Similar action may occur when ground meat is introduced into the intestinal tract. There the temperature is ideal for rapid spoilage. **This is particularly applicable if there is insufficient hydrochloric acid in the stomach**, as HCI acts as an intestinal antiseptic to inhibit fermentation and putrefaction which might otherwise occur. Here again, a proper digestive aid containing hydrochloric acid sources may be used to a distinct advantage.

NOTE: Preserved meats, such as weiners and sausages, do not have as much tendency to putrefaction, since they contain antiputrefactive chemicals (usually nitrites and/or nitrates) which work both inside and outside the body to produce this effect. However, for the same reason they are not desirable from a nutritional viewpoint. It has been determined that these substances inhibit enzymes in the body, produce liver and kidney disease, as well as being possibly carcinogenic.

Regarding the Use Of Sugar and Protein and/or Fat Combinations - One of the little known deleterious effects of refined sugar is its reaction in the gastrointestinal tract with protein and/or fat combinations. First of all, let us establish that concentrated carbohydrates (sugars) stay in the stomach for only a short period of time since very little digestion is necessary. On the other hand, protein remains in the stomach for extended periods of time (up to 5 hours) because much activity must take place before the proteins can be passed on to the small intestine for absorption. Some fats are also broken down in the stomach and the presence of fat in e stomach slows down the production of hydrochloric acid, which further delays the time of departure of stomach contents. When concentrated carbohydrates are mixed with protein/fat combinations, sugars tend to ferment in the stomach, producing gas. Adequate hydrochloric acid will prevent this to some extent, but the major cause of stomach gas is improper combining of food groups. Too many Americans are accustomed to finishing off a good protein meal with sweet desserts. For best nutrition, concentrated sweets should be eaten on an empty stomach, this includes fruits, fruit juices, etc., as well.

There are many sugar/protein combinations which may be easily avoided if one is on the alert; an outstanding example is eggs with orange juice. The fact that many food contain a combination of protein and carbohydrates must be taken into consideration - such natural combination rarely gives much trouble - as it is a concentration of carbohydrates which produces the deleterious effects, these being proportional to the quantity present.

Regarding the Use of Fiber Food in the Diet - As a natural laxative, without griping, diarrhea, or any of the other complaints we have about other laxatives, dietary fiber has no equal. Although many are not aware, they suffer from extremely slow movement of the digestive tract. There are many subsequences of such slow tract time:

1. Intestinal gas because of the fermentation of starches and sugars.

2. Diverticulosis due to the large amounts of fecal material pushing against the wall of the intestine, producing little sacs or pouches which then fill with waste material. This is ideal circumstances for more putrefaction to occur, which then discharges noxious matter into the tract which may be absorbed into the blood stream.

3. Hemorrhoids and varicosities can be blamed, at least in part, to the pressure exerted by the large amounts of material collected in the intestinal tract on the pelvic veins, creating back pressure which balloons the veins in the hemorrhoidal plexus and in the leg.

It would be a very apathetic individual indeed, who would not see the advantages of consuming some form of dietary fiber each and every day in order to help prevent the above from becoming a reality in his or her life. The Creative Restoration Diet suggests one-half cup of wheat, oat or corn bran flakes, usually found in health food stores. They can be mixed with granola, yogurt, salads, casseroles, etc. Bran or dietary fiber should not be referred to as "roughage" but rather as "softage" because it becomes very soft, water filled bulk in the intestines. The use of bran remedies the lack of fiber in a diet made up primarily of proteins (which contain very little fiber) and comparatively few raw fruits and vegetables.

Regarding the Use of Common Salt in the Diet - People who use as much salt as they like may excrete nine times as much potassium, an essential minerals, as those on salt restricted diets. Actually, Americans frequently consume 20 to 25 times as much salt as estimated sodium requirements recommend. If this is not counter-balanced with increased potassium intake, a borderline potassium deficiency state is easily brought about. Salt substitutes, mostly made up of potassium chloride, are often too bitter for anyone to stick with their use. We are fortunate in having a new 40-60 mixture of sodium and potassium chlorides and the minerals calcium and magnesium and kelp on the market. This satisfies flavor requirements and you need not worry about the loss of potassium from using sodium chloride alone. This formula is available in most health food stores.

OVERALL PICTURE OF THE CREATIVE RESTORATION DIET

In order to help you obtain a better idea of the recommended diet, examples of Desirable and Undesirable foods are listed. Of course, not all foods in each category can be shown, but a study of the examples given will suffice to show the type of food necessary for best results.

DESIRABLE FOODS

1. All Garden Vegetables (order of desirability - fresh, frozen, canned):

Asparagus	Tomato	Potatoes	Celery

Squash	Cauliflower	Garbanzas	Broccoli
Cabbage	Carrots	Parsley	Lettuce
Corn	String Beans	Rutabaga	Peas
Yams	Parsnips	Chard	Sprouts

2. Protein dishes (veal, beef, lamb, venison, elk, buffalo, fish, eggs, cheese):
   Meats should be broiled
   Cheese should be unprocessed

3. Fermented Foods
   Buttermilk, Yogurt, Cottage cheese, Sauerkraut

4. Fruits, Fruit Juices, Vegetable Juices
   All are acceptable - just be careful as to the combinations of fruits and/or fruit juices with proteins.

5. Nuts and Seeds
   These are preferable in the raw state or dry roasted with little salt. They belong to the protein/fat category of foods.

6. Dietary Fiber
   Wheat Bran, Rice Bran, Oat Bran, Pectin

UNDESIRABLE FOODS

1. Commercially Processed Flour Products
   White Breads, White Buns, Biscuits, White Rolls, Doughnuts, Cookies, Cakes, Pie Crusts

2. Commercially Processed White Sugar Products

Pie, Candy, Cakes, Pudding, Soda Pop, Doughnuts

3. Processed or Ground Meat
   Hamburger, Meat Loaf, Weiners, Sausage, Hash, Lunch Meats, Potted Meats, Chili
   (The exception to ground meat is when you grind it fresh and immediately use it.)

4. Sugar - Protein Combinations
   Ice Cream, Chocolate Milk, Milk Shakes, Baked Beans, Fruits or Fruit Juices with meat, eggs, cheese, Desserts with meals

LIVER-KIDNEY-BOWEL CLEANSING DIET

One of the most important factors in any disease conditions is the detoxification of the body. It should also follow that such a detoxification can be an excellent means of preventing disease and promoting good health. The following is a simple three day program which accomplishes detoxification of the major organs involved in retaining toxins in the body:

Materials Needed:

1. From 12 to 16 lemons daily, depending on size. (If fresh lemons are unavailable, you can buy pure concentrated lemon juice.)
2. From 2 to 3 quarts of distilled water daily.
3. Small amount of honey.
4. One bottle of an herb combination containing garlic, mandrake, quassia, black cohosh, chaparral, fenugreek, red sage, and goldenseal.

5. One bottle of dietary fiber tablets.
   (May be called bran tablets.)

FIRST DAY: One and one-half cups freshly squeezed (or the equivalent of concentrate) lemon juice mixed with two quarts of distilled water and a little honey for palatability. This will be your total intake of fluid and food for the day, so you may sip on it constantly. Take 2 of the herb tablets both morning and evening. Take 8 dietary fiber tablets in the morning and 8 in the afternoon, with a ten ounce glass of lemon mixture.

SECOND DAY: Repeat the mixing of the approximately 2 1/2 quarts of lemon juice-distilled water-honey mixture and consume it during the day. Use 3 of the herb tablets morning and evening and 8 dietary fiber tablets twice daily.

THIRD DAY: Repeat the mixing of the approximately 2 1/2 quarts of lemon juice-distilled water-honey mixture and consume it during the day. Use 4 of the herb tablets morning and evening and 8 dietary fiber tablets twice daily.

This is the end of the concentrated detoxifying, but the first week after this program is extremely important, regarding the lasting benefits. The following suggestions as to eating should be observed:

FOURTH AND FIFTH DAY: Stop using the lemon juice-distilled water-honey mixture, but continue the use of 2 herb tablets morning and evening. Also, use 8 dietary fiber tablets morning and afternoon. Drink all you wish of tomato juice, carrot juice, grape juice (dilute the grape juice with about one-third spring water) or other vegetable or fruit juices. Eliminate citrus juices. Consume all the fresh spring water you wish.

SIXTH AND SEVENTH DAY: Add raw fruits and vegetables to your regime, maintaining herb and dietary fiber tablet intake as before. Consume all the fresh juices that you wish.

EIGHTH DAY: Add yogurt and/or cottage cheese, continue dietary fiber and herb tablets twice daily as before.

NINTH DAY: Add lightly steamed vegetables to allowable foods. Reduce dietary fiber tablets to 12 daily, and continue taking 4 herb tablets on a daily basis.

TENTH DAY: If desired, add small portion of meat to one meal - seeds, nuts or eggs are just as acceptable. Reduce dietary fiber tablets to 4 in the morning and 4 in the afternoon, and continue taking 4 herb tablets daily.

ELEVENTH DAY FORWARD: Follow the Creative Restoration Diet; adjust dietary fiber tablets according to personal need. Lower bowel gas and foul odored stools are indications of increased need for dietary fiber. You may now discontinue the herb tablets.

OTHER USES OF HERBS

Taking herbs by mouth, either in tablet or capsule form, or as a tincture or tea are by far the most popular ways of using herbs. We should not overlook the exquisite ways that herbs can be used externally.

HERBAL BATHS - A warm, leisurely bath has long found favor as a relaxing and tension easing experience. But the warm water can be improved upon both from a cleansing viewpoint as well as the delightful fragrances one can achieve very simply. Try putting a handful of dried mint and a handful of thyme in a nylon sock. Make sure your tap water is very hot and let the hot water run over the bag for a couple of minutes, then fill the tub with the desired temperature of water. Step in and expect a most relaxing and delightfully scented respite.

For skin rejuvenation, try a mixture of comfrey, alfalfa, parsley, and orange peel. This will help almost all kinds of skin problems, if used faithfully.

Chamomile and sage leaves are excellent for sore, aching muscles, just use a handful of each in the nylon sock and tie it off. Then you can use the bag to massage your muscles while in the bath.

AROMATIC (HERBAL) WATERS. . . . You ladies can make your own sweet smelling splashes very simply, using only natural ingredients. (The list of ingredients on most commercial preparations should be incentive.) Lemon Water: Take either fresh or dried lemon leaves, place them in an enamel pot, cover with distilled water and slowly bring to a boil. Simmer for several minutes, strain and presto - you have it! Rose Water: Use the identical procedure as above except use rose petals; orange leaves and blossoms, clover and many other can be prepared this same way.

HOMEOPATHY

Homeopathy was discovered by the German physician Dr. Samuel Hahnemann in the early 1800's. Dr. Hahnemann had been disillusioned with the medical practice at that time because he felt that the medical treatment he learned and studied addressed the symptoms that the person was displaying, and never dealt with the underlying cause of the problem. None of the medicines that he gave ever facilitated the body's own healing process, nor did they help the person really become well. He felt that he was strictly practicing patchwork medicine, making a person feel better until the body could heal itself. Intuitively, Dr. Hahnemann knew that a medicine did exist that could help the body get well. A medicine could work with the body in a team effort to strengthen and speed up the healing process, assisting the body's ability to overcome illness that it could not alone overcome.

THE BEGINNING

It was in pursuit of this new form of non-injurious medicine that Dr. Hahnemann devoted ten years of his life to medical research until finally his first successful experience occurred; Dr. Hahnemann treated a malaria patient with homeopathic quinine.

The homeopathic dose of this very potent drug stimulated the person's immune system and boosted it much in the way a battery boosts a car that is dead. This boost to the immune system was strong enough for the body to kill the parasites that caused the disease of malaria. This increased immune respone allowed the cause to be eliminated and the person became well. Dr. Hahnemann experienced a cure for malaria.

From this point, Dr. Hahnemann began treating illnesses successfully and, during an epidemic of typhoid fever in Germany, Dr. Hahnemann had the highest cure rate of any physician using his homeopathic medicines. This brought a great interest in homeopathy. Many of Dr. Hahnemann's colleagues chose to study with him. Homeopathic medicine spread throughout Germany, France, England, and Europe itself. Homeopathy moved into Asia, India and even into the United States. By 1840, twenty to forty percent of all doctors in America were homeopathic physicians. In the early 1900's, the first president of the FDA was a homeopathic physician. Then came the first of the so-called "miracle drugs" - penicillin. Penicillin had a profound effect on "modern" medicine. Doctors believed that soon the world would be free of all disease through the use of potent drugs.

An entire category of drugs was formed called OTC - "over the counter" drugs. The pharmaceutical companies began producing a greater variety of drugs; and with this illusion of a miracle cure. . . .just pop the pill and become well. . . .Homeopathy was overlooked by the public. Then in 1960, thalidomide caused birth defects, they cyclamates caused cancer. Birth control pills were found to cause high blood pressure, and people became more wary of the drugs they were taking. Drugs are now considered potentially dangerous. Even aspirin is found to cause gastric bleeding and immune system repression and carries warnings with its use. Now in the 1990's, we realize there has been no miracle. Disease is more rampant than ever before, and the need for a medicine that truly works with your body, without toxic side effects, is needed. To fill this need, homeopathy has re-emerged.

HOW DOES HOMEOPATHIC MEDICINE WORK?

To understand homeopathic medicine, you must understand how the body functions. Your body has evolved from just a single fertilized cell to some sixty trillion cells. Every cell of your body has a specific function to perform. It repairs and maintains itself in what is a perfect harmony of your body's vital functions. Homeostatic balance is a perfect harmony of your body's vital functions. Your body is able to maintain this homeostatic balance under all conditions, such as stress, poor diet, even illness in people around you. Illness which you can usually successfully fight off by delivering strength to your own immune system.

HOMEOSTATIC IMBALANCE

Then one time in a thousand you are impacted by some pathogen that your defense system cannot protect you from. This impact throws your body out of homeostatic balance. As soon as this imbalance occurs, your body immediately goes to work trying to offset and overcome this pathogen. Your immune system is trying to bring your body back into a state of balance. As your body is alerted and tries to fight this invading agent, your blood flow and nerve force to the area increases. Your body generates symptoms while the battle is being fought. These symptoms indicate where your body needs strength and indicates the stage of the battle. To a homeopathic physician, these symptoms tell him exactly what type of medicines to use a stimulate the body in exactly the right location, with the right amount of strength to boost the body's own natural healing process, and to boost it with enough strength to overcome the cause of the illness and bring back the homeostatic balance.

Conventional medicine recognizes homeostatic balance and recognizes that the balance of this homeostatic balance is essential. Conventional medicine also recognizes that when the homeostatic balance is upset, the person becomes ill. However, at this point, the conventional form of medicine chooses to use drugs to alleviate the suffering from the symptoms. Drugs do nothing to stimulate and assist the body's own healing process so, at best, the body is made less miserable. You suffer less, but your body still must heal itself before you are able to get well. All the drugs do is make the suffering easier and suppress the symptoms. If you body continues to fight and lose, fight and lose, your body becomes tired. If your body fights at a lesser intensity and the offending agent seeps deeper into your body, it may create a more chronic imbalance. The symptoms have diminished only because your body can no longer fight, and a weakening effect occurs. This is the sad case of drug therapy.

Homeopathic philosophy says that the only reason your body can become ill is if the strength of your body's ability to heal itself is diminished. The stimulation with homeopathic medicines coordinates the vital force in your body and gives you greater resistance. Your body, with its own power restored, can throw off the cause of the illness and you become well. In homeopathic medicines, when the symptoms go away, the body has overcome the cause of the illness and with balance restored, the body is well!

WHAT IS HOMEOPATHIC MEDICINE?

Homeopathic medicine is extracted from a plant, mineral or animal substance and made into medicine by a process called potentization. This medicine is given in minute doses and stimulates the body to respond and fight. The stimulation acts very much the way a vaccination acts in the body. A small dose of a potent medicine stimulates the immune system into activity, and with this increased activity, the body destroys the attacking agent and you become well. The results of homeopathic medical treatment are: increased vitality, an increase in your overall state of health, and the elimination of the causative agents that create an imbalance in your body. Homeopathy has the ability to heal and repair. A common result of conventional drug therapy is chronic illness. Today, there is more chronic disease than ever before in history, and yet more money is spent on medical research; there are more hospitals, more doctors, more drugs and more forms of medical therapy than ever before on this planet.

What can be done to bring back health? What can a person do to improve their overall state of health? There are only two medical systems that have this ability. One system is acupuncture. Acupuncture was recently introduced into the United States. In the beginning, "orthodox" doctors felt that acupuncture was a great Chinese placebo, and they made light of this 4,000 year old system of medicine. However, with time and clinical experiments and double blind studies, acupuncture has proven effective as a form of medicine. Acupuncture was so effective that doctors have incorporated it into their medical license. Acupuncture has reached full status as a medical healing art.

The other system of medicine is homeopathy. In fact, the only two official compendium of licensed medicine in the United States are the United States Pharmacopoeia, which contains a listing of all drugs allowed to be used by doctors in drug therapy, and the Homeopathic Pharmacopoeia of the United States which lists the official medical therapy. As an example of how homeopathic medicine helps to heal and repair, let's assume we have a person who knows they have a bad liver, and it just doesn't function like it did when they were young. The patient asks the doctor, "What can you do for me?" The doctor will say, "All I can do is tell you how to let the body recover on its own."

No drug has ever been invented that can heal or repair the

liver, and no drug the doctor has to offer can give that patient a better liver. The patient who goes to his homeopathic doctor and asks for help for his liver gets a different approach. The homeopathic doctor gives the patient a series of homeopathic medicines that stimulate the body's own liver maintenance system. The body is always trying to repair the liver, all it needs is greater energy to overcome the problem. The homeopathic medicine provides this energy, and the body, with this help, restores the liver back to health.

FIVE TYPES OF HOMEOPATHY

There are five types of homeopathic medical treatments. The first type of homeopathic treatment is the use of singular remedies. This generally requires a trained homeopathic physician. This physician takes an extensive history of all the symptoms that are present and, by understanding the full totality of the symptoms a person is displaying, choose the one best homeopathic medicine to fit the total response the body has to this imbalance; that medicine is usually given in a strong potency. The process of the repair and restoration of health is watched closely by the homeopathic physician, and at a certain point, a new medicine will be given. This process is repeated, and the patient is watched closely until normal health is restored. The use of these singular remedies and the skill of the homeopathic physician, combined with the use of higher potencies, make this ultimately a bit more tedious than most patients will endure unless they have tried other methods for a long time.

Another form of homeopathic therapy is the use of tissue salts. Tissue salts are a subset of homeopathic remedies developed by Dr. Schuessler in Germany. Dr. Schuessler studied the intracellular chemistry of the body because he felt that if he could understand how to make the single cells of the body healthy, the whole body could be made well. In his study, Dr. Schuessler found twelve minerals salts that must maintain a specific balance with each other in the cells of the body. He also found that if these salts were in balance properly, the person was healthy and not susceptible to an illness. However, if one or more of these salts were out of balance, a certain susceptibility pattern would start to manifest and Dr. Schuessler could predict, from the salt that was out of balance, what this pattern of susceptibility would be and what the pattern of illness was likely to become. By giving the homeopathic tissue salt, Dr. Schuessler was able to restore the normal cellular balance and break the pattern of susceptibility the person was displaying and bring them back to health. So the use of tissue salts helps break chronic patterns of susceptibility. You don't need to be ill to take a tissue salt. You may be the kind of person who has chronic difficulty with water retention, or you may always get a cold in the chest whenever you become ill. Or, you may be the type of person who gets chronic indigestion. It is these chronic patterns of susceptability that the tissue salts are excellent at bringing back into balance and repairing.

Another form of homeopathic treatment is the use of homeopathic glandular and organ products called organo therapy. These homeopathic glands and organs stimulate a similar gland in your body. If you take homeopathic adrenal gland, the substance will stimulate your adrenal glands into greater activity and greater health. Homeopathic liver extracts will stimulate the vital functions of your liver. It will help your liver improve its overall well being and increase its capacity to regain its state of health. Since 1930, homeopathic organo therapy has taken its place as a major branch of homeopathic medicine. These homeopathic gland and organ products give you another way of working on your body, so you can tune up your organs and tune up your endocrine system. If you are under a great deal of stress, you can work on your adrenal glands. If you have blood sugar imbalances, you can work on your pancreas. If you have chronic problems with weight, you can work on your thyroid. These products work by coordinating and stimulating your own vitality in that given gland or an organ, and your health is gained by a return to homeostatic balance. You cannot over-stimulate a gland or an organ with this homeopathic medicine, you can only bring it back to health by bringing back its normal function.

HOMEOPATHIC COMBINATIONS

The fourth type of homeopathic treatment is the use of homeopathic formulas made from combinations of homeopathic medicines found in Homeopathic Pharmacopoeia. These combinations represent the greatest breakthrough for homeopathy. An effective formula can be made for an illness, and a person can treat himself homeopathically. This combination of ingredients coordinates and energizes the body's response to an illness and rapidly brings a person back to health. These combinations have the name of the illnesses they treat on the label and have finally given homeopathic medicine the ability to put "over the counter" products on the market to give people a real choice in their medical treatment. With modern technology, combinations have become extremely effective; they now represent three-fourths of all the homeopathic treatments used in the world today.

The fifth type of homeopathic treatment is the use of combination formulas topically for skin infections. The skin is the largest organ of the body and performs many crucial functions essential to health. Now homeopathic ointments are available to treat the many illnesses that occur on the skin.

PRODUCTION OF A HOMEOPATHIC REMEDY

In preparing a homeopathic remedy, an organic product, usually an herb, is selected and the active medicinal ingredient is removed. This is usually accomplished with an alcohol extraction, using other adjuncts such as grinding, macerating, applying heat, etc., to accomplish the end result -- a concentrated active ingredient.

Next, a given quantity of this active substance is diluted with nine parts of water and alcohol and vigorously mixed. This mixing is called potentization and the resulting mixture is called a 1X potency.

One part of this 1X solution is put into nine parts of water and alcohol and is again violently shaken or potentized. This solution is stronger in its medical power than the 1X, and is called 2X. One part of this 2X solution is again put into nine parts of water and alcohol and violently shaken. This potency is called 3X; and this process can continue to a 6X, 12X, 60X, 200X, even to a 10,000X or 50,000X potency.

It has been found that each time the medicine is potentized, the medicine becomes stronger and works at a deeper level in the body. The higher potencies are so much stronger than the 50,000X medicines are only given once in a person's lifetime. For a long time, the understanding of diluting and potentizing did not make sense to pharmacologists. There is no way to understand how this potentizing process could make a medicine more active. However, modern physics, with Albert Einstein's equation - $E = MC^2$ - gives us an explanation. This equation states that as matter is reduced, large amounts of energy are released. The first proof of this equation was the atom bomb; the more matter that was reduced, the more energy was released. Thus, physics gives us an understanding of homeopathic medicine. The energy in the homeopathic medicine, in addition to the energy of the body's own system of healing and repair, combines to restore the state of balance. As these medicines are diluted and potentized, diluted and potentized, you go from a 1X to a 2X, to a 3X, and soon you reach the level of 24X potency. At a 24X potency, modern chemists say that there are no more molecules of the original medically active substance present, and that any potency higher than a 24X could not be effective. For a long time, chemists have said a modern piece of analytical equipment called an x-ray fluorescence detection device can now show a complete and accurate spectrum of the medically active substance in a solution that is beyond a 24X potency. This proves that the pattern of energy remains, even though there are no molecules of the original medically active substance present.

ARE HOMEOPATHIC MEDICINES SAFE?

There have been no known poisonings from the use of homeopathic medicine in its entire history, nor are there any known side effects. Homeopathic medicine is safe for children, the elderly, people who are very allergic, pregnant women and women who are nursing; in fact, homeopathy represents the safest form of effective medicine known.

HOW DO WE KNOW HOMEOPATHIC MEDICINES ARE EFFECTIVE?

The greatest test of efficacy that science has ever demonstrated is in clinical evidence. Homeopathy has 180 years of clinical evidence. There are homeopathic physicians who go to medical school and, after they graduate, go back to school for four more years to train as a homeopath. There are homeopathic hospitals, and double blind tests of homeopathic medicines that have been done on humans and animals. Double blind tests have been conducted to show how homeopathic mercury removes mercury from the body. Homeopathic lead removes lead from the body. Homeopathic arsenic removes arsenic from the body. These tests show that homeopathic medicine can do what no known drugs are able to do. Many times a person will ask, "Can I take a homeopathic medicine and still use the drugs my doctor has given me?" The answer is yes. Drugs given under the care of a physician can have a very powerful effect in regulating the chemistry of the body, and in certain emergency cases, these drugs could be invaluable in saving lives. But with drug therapy, the body still must heal itself. So homeopathy is medicine given to stimulate the body's own healing process and can aid tremendously in the overall approach a person takes to getting well. There has been no known drug interaction between a homeopathic medicine and an orthodox drug.

Homeopathic treatment also improves with good nutrition. Your body is made up of vitamins and minerals and amino acids. It is essential that a person who is interested in health be aware that the food taken into the body ultimately becomes part of the body. If you take food into your body that is full of chemicals, full of preservatives, full of dyes, your chemistry will become affected. Your body will be forced to fight the battle of balance every day, every time you eat. Sooner or later, you body will become tired. Your liver will be unable to handle any more poison and your kidneys will become too irritated to work effectively. Nutrition is very, very important. Foods that have been grown organically, vitamins that are made from natural processes and amino acids isolated and crystallized can give the body the building blocks necessary for health.

HOW FAST CAN HOMEOPATHIC MEDICINES WORK?

They work very quickly. In fact, as soon as they are put under the tongue, they go into your system. As the stimulation begins, your body responds. The length of time for the elimination of the symptoms depends on the individual, because the medicine is working with your body to overcome the causes of the imbalances for the condition of your body. The condition of your vitality determines how fast the medicine will work. If you are strong and vital, the results can be immediate, but if you are chronically ill, the results may take days but, you will get the results.

What is a total homeopathic health program? For a total homeopathic treatment a person can take a combination or a formula for an illness, a tissue salt for the susceptibility to the illness, and a glandular product or an organ product to support the body's recovery, and these can be taken all at the same time. In the case where a battle has just begun and the fight is raging, you can take the homeopathic medicine very often, up to every half hour. As you take this medicine every half hour, you will improve the body's capacity to get well, so that the acute stage passes very quickly. If you are working on a chronic imbalance that has been there a long time, you should take the homeopathic medicine at a lower frequency, two times a day or four times a day. You want to boost the body and let the body respond, and again boost the body and let it respond. As the body's response gets stronger, you can begin taking the homeopathic medicine more often, until the person goes through the complete healing process.

WHAT IS CELL PLASMA?

Cell plasma is a combination of all twelve tissue salts and is used as a general cell nutrient, much in the way a multiple vitamin would be used for the body's overall health. The cell plasma taken regularly can help maintain the balance of all the cells in the body. A multiple gland and organ product similarly will stimulate the overall endocrine system of your body and maintain general good vitality and health.

THE CELL SALTS

In the days gone by, classical homeopaths used a great deal of care in selecting the correct and specific remedy. There was a belief that homeopathic remedies counteracted one another and the use of a very specific remedy was the only way to use these remedies. Today, with years of use and experience to guide us, modern thinking feels that the use of combination homeopathic cell salts in the form of a single tincture may be the best practice, especially as a preventive.

BIOPLASMA is such a combination and has become one of the most popular of all the cell salt medications.

The formula includes:

Calcarea fluorica (Calc. Fluor.)
Calcarea phosphorica (Calc. phos.)
Calcarea sulfate (Calc. sulf.)
Ferrum phosphoricum (Ferrum phos.)
Kali muriaticum (Kali mur.)
Kali phosphoricum (Kali phos.)
Kali sulfuricum (Kali sulf.)
Magnesium phosphoricum (Mag. phos.)
Natrium muriaticum (Nat. mur.)
Natrium phosphoricum (Nat. phos.)
Natrium sulfuricum (Nat. sulf.)

This combination cell salt formula is considered by many modern homeopathic as a quick general remedy, particularly when other indications are not clear. Also as a general addition to any other homeopathic remedy in use. Thus, BIOPLASMA has many uses in the area of natural healing.

ORGAN AND GLANDULAR TINCTURES

Organs such as the stomach, heart, kidneys, liver, and lungs perform many important functions such as the digestion of our food intake, circulation and purification of our blood, and the exchange of waste carbon dioxide for life and energy producing oxygen. Glands such as the pituitary, thyroid, pancreas, adrenals, thymus and spleen and sex glands are part of the endocrine system producing hormones that stimulate and inhibit organ functions.

It has been our experience that all the organs and glands work in such a synchronous fashion that it is usually not beneficial to work with isolated units, but instead to combine them all together into two formulae - one for the female and one for the male. Such combinations contain homeopathic dilutions of all the organs and glands, prepared from non-commercial cattle that have not been fed antibiotics and were allowed to roam the range, instead of being confined and literally force-fed. These organs and glands are freeze dried, preventing the possibility of deterioration and/or contamination. The freeze dried extracts are then combined and this material is now processed as any other homeopathic preparation with continual dilution until the desired potency is reached.

Since the concept of healthy organs and glands is such a basic ingredient for good health, it only makes sense that the individual would be very interested in the structural rehabilitation of these organs and glands. Homeopathic dilutions are one of the methods of reactivating tissues, wherever they may be; so it might behoove you to consider the possibility of the use of one of the following homeopathic glandular formulas.

Male Multi-Gland & Organ		Female Multi-Gland & Organ	
Duodenal	Thyroid	Duodenal	Thyroid
Lung	Thymus	Lung	Thymus
Heart	Orchic	Heart	Ovary
Kidney	Prostate	Kidney	Adrenal
Adrenal			

These are alcohol tinctures and should be used under the tongue, 10 drops two to four times daily.

LIQUIDS VS. TABLETS

How do liquids compare to homeopathic lactose tablets? The use of a liquid homeopathic is recommended over homeopathic medicines in a lactose based tablet, and this occurs for two reasons. In traditional homeopathic therapy, you are cautioned not to drink coffee, eat garlic, drink peppermint tea, or eat any food that has strong odors during the course of the treatment. This is because strong odors can affect the homeopathic medicine that is made in sugar lactose tablets. Homeopathic medicines made in alcohol, however, are not subject to deterioration by these strong foods, and the homeopathic medicine and the alcohol then forms the most resistant form of homeopathic medicine that a consumer can buy. Often there is a concern, especially for children and reformed alcoholics. This alcohol can be evaporated if drops of the medicine are placed into a cup of boiling water, the alcohol evaporates, and you then sip the medicated water, just as you would sip tea.

Do homeopathic medicines deteriorate with age? Homeopathic medicines, especially medicines made in an alcohol solution, last indefinitely. An expiration date is required by the FDA on all medicines. The expiration date does not indicate the medicine will deteriorate at that point of time, but only how old the product is, and it serves as a reminder for the retailer to continue updating and rotating the stock. There has been no proof, ever, that a medicine only lasts three years or five years in an alcohol solution.

IN SUMMARY

Homeopathic medicine represents that most interesting system of healing and repairing the body that exists today; homeopathy is recognized the world over. It is a system that has an official compendium authorized by the government and is a system now available to help knowledgeable people in the United States make a choice between natural medicines to boost the body's own natural healing process, or chemical drugs such aspirin, Nyquil, Clearasil and Contact, which suppress the symptoms and leave the cause of the illness untouched.

Homeopathic medicines are in virtually every health food store in the country. Now you have an opportunity to experience good health, to regain the vitality that you have lost and to realize that the greatest physician in the world is your own body. Learn how to help it, and enjoy good health.

The *Dr. Donsbach Tells You* Series
28 Titles Covering a Wide Variety of Topics

Arthritis
Acne, Eczema, Psoriasis
Acupressure & Reflex Massage
Alfalfa, Bee Pollen & Ginseng
Allergies, Stress & Asthma
Benign Prostatic Hypertrophy & Prostate Cancer
Blood & Urine Tests Explained
Cancer (Wholistic Therapy)
Candidiasis & Chronic Fatigue Syndrome
Cataracts & Glaucoma
Embracing Wholistic Health
Get Well & Stay Well Through Detoxification
Heart Disease, Stroke, Oral & Intravenous Chelation
High Blood Pressure
Homeopathy & Herbs
Indigestion, Ulcers, Colitis & Constipation
Live Cell Therapy
Multiple Sclerosis, Muscular Dystrophy & ALS
Non-Invasive Testing
Overweight & Underweight
Oxygen, Oxygen, Oxygen
PMS, Menopause & Hysterectomy
Saturated & Unsaturated Fats (EPA & GLA)
SOD, DLPA, GLA & DMSO
Vitamins, Minerals and Amino Acids
Water

NOTES:

NOTES:

NOTES:

NOTES:

NOTES:

NOTES:

NOTES: